Keto Cocktails 2021

Tasty Keto Friendly Alcohol Drinks for Beginners you Can Make at Home for Your Friends and Family

Jenny Kern

Table Of Contents

Introduction

Thank you for purchasing this keto cocktail book. There are some recipes in this book that will ask you to make something along the lines of "mix with ice". In these recipes, you pour all the ingredients into a blender and then put the ice on and blend until you get a smooth, even consistency. Crushed ice works best for these recipes as it makes the job a lot easier on the blender. In this book you will also find other techniques to make the best of your favorite drinks, and I am sure that over time you will learn them perfectly by becoming a true expert in DIY cocktails. Enjoy.

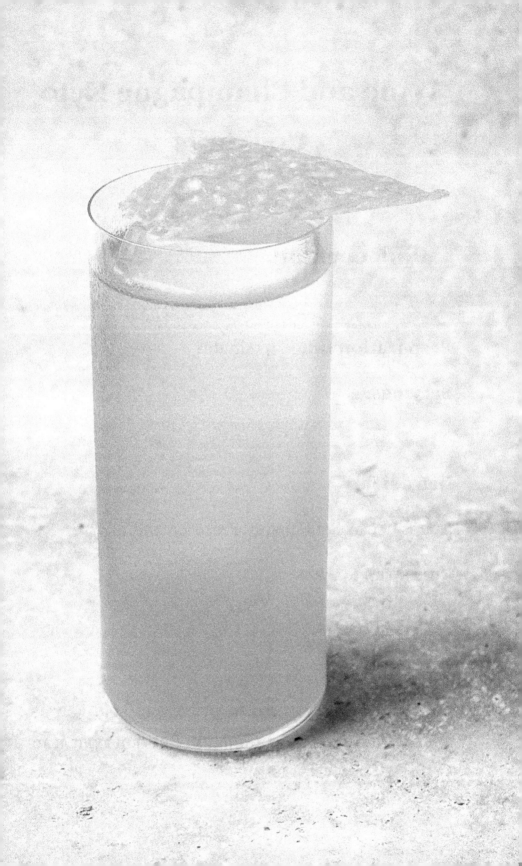

Wine and Champagne Keto Cocktails

Pink cocktail

Preparation time: 5 minutes

Servings: 2

Ingredients:

2 cups of excellent quality Prosecco, or Cartizze

Rose syrup to taste

Directions:

First of all the Prosecco must be very cold and as already said of excellent quality. But don't put it in the freezer, cool it in the ice bucket, or put it in the refrigerator for a while.

Pour the Prosecco into the two glasses, then slowly pour a spoonful of rose syrup into each.

Let the syrup settle on the bottom without mixing, obtaining a beautiful decorative effect.

Serve immediately on a tray that you can decorate with rose petals or with a flower.

Godly Sangria

Preparation time: 10 minutes

Servings: 7

Ingredients:

¼ cup vanilla syrup (such as Monin)

½ cup black cherries, pitted and cut in half

¾ cup coconut rum

1 bottle dry white wine

1 cup pineapple chunks

1 orange, cut into half-wheels

1 peach, pitted and cut

7-Up, as required (not necessary)

Directions:

Mix all of the ingredients apart from the 7-Up in a big ceramic or glass container and stir thoroughly.

Cover and place in your fridge for a minimum of 4 hours (preferably overnight).

Serve over ice.

Grape Blast Sangria

Preparation time: 10 minutes

Servings: 12

Ingredients:

¼ cup sugar

½ cup green grapes, cut in half

½ cup red seedless grapes, cut in half

1 bottle dry white wine (pinot grigio or sauvignon blanc)

1 cup white grape juice

1 lemon, cut into wheels

1 lime, cut into wheels

1 liter 7 -Up

1 orange, cut into wheels

Directions:

Mix all of the ingredients apart from the 7-Up in a big ceramic or glass container and stir thoroughly until sugar dissolves.

Cover and place in your fridge for a minimum of 4 hours (preferably overnight).

Just before you serve, put in the 7-Up.

Serve over ice.

Hibiscus Sangria

Preparation time: 15 minutes

Servings: 5

Ingredients:

¼ cup Hendricks gin

¼ cup orange curaçao

½ cup lemon juice

½ cup Simple Syrup (page 6)

1 bottle dry white wine

1 lemon, cut

1 liter 7-Up

1 orange, cut

2 cups hibiscus tea (already steeped and cooled)

orchids, for decoration

thin lemon wheels

Directions:

Mix all of the ingredients apart from the 7-Up and garnishes in a big ceramic or glass container and stir thoroughly.

Cover and place in your fridge for a minimum of 4 hours.

Serve over ice; fill glasses about half full, then top with 7-Up.

Decorate using a floating lemon wheel and an orchid.

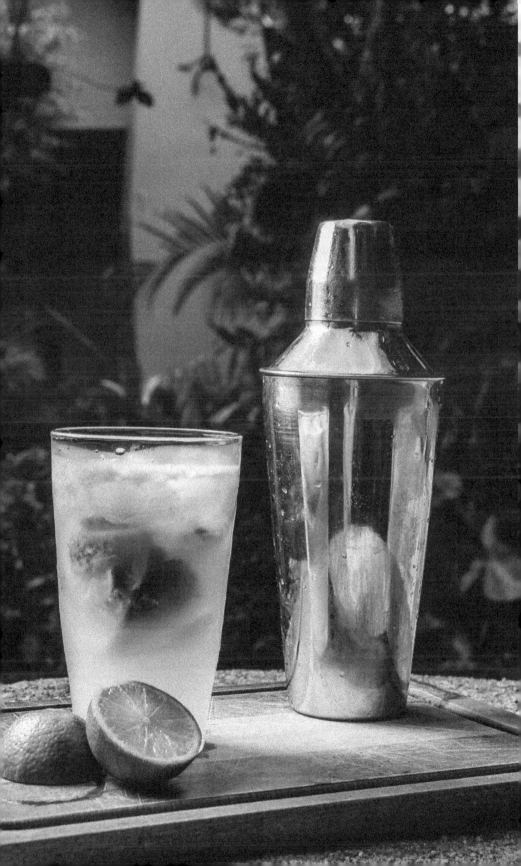

Gin Keto Cocktails

Bronx

Preparation time: 5 minutes

Servings: 3

Ingredients:

1 oz. gin

½ oz. red vermouth

½ oz. dry vermouth

¾ oz. orange juice

Ice

Directions:

Pour ¾ oz. of orange juice, ½ oz. of red vermouth, ½ oz. of dry vermouth, and 1 oz. of gin into a shaker

Fill the shaker with ice cubes and shake then strain

Dry Martini

Preparation time: 5 minutes

Servings: 2

Ingredients:

2 ½ oz. gin

½ oz. dry vermouth Martini

Ice

Green olives, for garnish

Directions:

Pour ½ oz. of dry vermouth and 2 ½ oz. of gin into a mixing glass

Fill the glass with ice cubes and stir gently

Garnish with a green olive on a cocktail skewer after straining in a chilled glass

Gimlet

Preparation time: 3 minutes

Servings: 1

Ingredients:

2 oz. gin

1 oz. lime juice

Ice

Lime zest, for garnish

Directions:

Pour 1 oz. of lime juice and 2 oz. of gin into a shaker

Fill the shaker with ice cubes and shake

Garnish with lime zest after straining in a chilled glass

Gin and Tonic

Preparation time: 5 minutes

Servings: 2

Ingredients:

1½ oz. gin

5 oz. tonic

Ice

Lime, for garnish

Directions:

Fill a highball glass to the top with ice

Pour in 1½ oz. of gin

Top up with tonic and stir gently

Garnish with 2 lime wheels

Martinez

Preparation time: 5 minutes

Servings: 2

Ingredients:

1 oz. gin

1 oz. red vermouth

¼ oz. Maraschino liqueur

Orange bitters

Orange zest

Ice

Directions:

Pour ¼ oz. of Maraschino liqueur, 1 oz. of red vermouth, and 1 oz. of gin into a mixing glass

Add 1 dash of orange bitters

Fill the glass with ice cubes and stir gently

Squeeze orange zest over the glass and put into the cocktail after straining in a chilled glass

Caraway Cantaloupe Gin

Preparation time: 15 minutes

Servings: 5

Ingredients:

175 to 350ml dry gin

1 ripe cantaloupe, peeled and balled or finely chopped

1 tablespoon caraway seeds, lightly bruised with a mortar and pestle

Directions:

Place all ingredients in a sealable glass container. Seal and shake to mix.

Set aside in a cool, dark location for 2 to 3 weeks. Check on taste periodically. Shake more for more flavor.

Strain out the solids and rebottle the newly infused gin.

Serve with a tonic and a piece of cantaloupe for garnish.

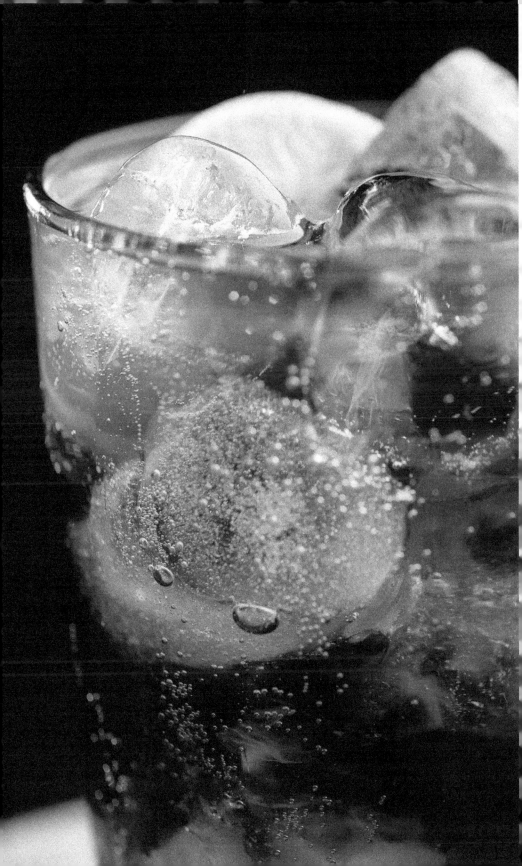

Whiskey Keto Cocktails

Sour, New York Style

Preparation time: 10 minutes

Servings: 1

Ingredients:

50ml whiskey, rye whiskey works best with this cocktail

2 tsp maple syrup

25ml fresh lemon juice

A dash of bitter orange

20ml red wine

1 tbsp egg white

A handful of ice cubes

Directions:

Take a cocktail shaker and add the whiskey, maple syrup, orange bitters, and lemon juice

Place the egg white onto a small plate and stir quickly with a spoon to loosen up

Pour the egg white into the shaker and shake

Add some ice cubes and shake once more, until the outside feels cold

Take your serving glass and strain the mixture inside, leaving a little space at the top

Fill up the rest of the glass with the red wine

After a couple of seconds, the wine will float to just underneath where the frothy section is (the egg white)

Manhattan Whiskey

Preparation time: 5 minutes

Servings: 1

Ingredients:

50ml bourbon

25ml vermouth (Rosso is best)

2 dashes of Angostura bitters

A handful of ice cubes

5ml cherry syrup (from a jar of maraschino cherries)

1 maraschino cherry for decoration

A twist of lemon for decoration

Directions:

Take a mixing jug and add all the ingredients, apart from the decorations

Combine gently with a bar spoon

Use a strainer to pour into your serving glass

Add the cherry and twist of lemon on top for decoration

Creamy Bourbon

Preparation time: 5 minutes

Servings: 2

Ingredients:

4 tbsp creme de cacao

4 tbsp fresh lemon juice

4 tbsp bourbon

4 tsp caster sugar

A handful of ice cubes

A little orange zest for decoration

Directions:

Take a cocktail shaker and combine all the ingredients

Shake to combine, until the outside of the shaker is cold

Take two martini glasses and pour the cocktail inside

Decorate with zest and serve

Traditional Irish whiskey

Preparation time: 5 minutes

Servings: 1

Ingredients:

10ml Sauternes

40ml Irish whiskey

10ml elderflower (cordial)

A handful of ice cubes

A little lemon zest for decoration

Directions:

Add the ingredients to a mixing jug

Use a bar spoon to carefully coming everything together

Make sure the ice cubes have melted slightly before serving

Pour into your cocktail glass

Garnish with a little lemon zest for decoration

Whiskey Punch

Preparation time: 10 minutes

Servings: 6

Ingredients:

1 3/4 cups Irish whiskey

1/4 cup (packed) golden brown sugar

6 thick lemon slices

24 whole cloves

3 cups hot water

Directions:

In a pitcher, combine sugar and whiskey until the sugar has dissolved. Split the mixture among 6 heat-proof glasses.

Use 4 cloves to stud in per lemon slice then put each one in a glass.

Add a half cup of hot water into each and finish by stirring to combine all.

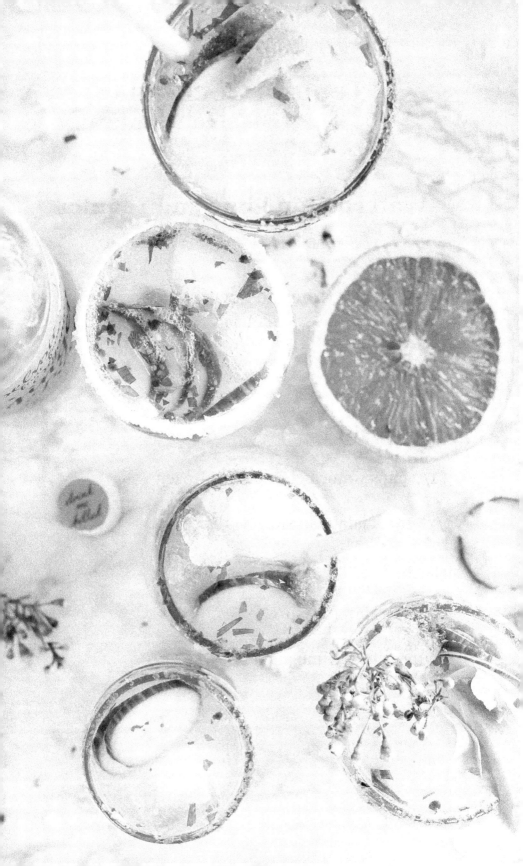

Tequila Cocktails

Watermelon Lime and Tequila

Preparation time: 10 minutes

Servings: 6

Ingredients:

3 1/2 cups watermelon pieces, frozen

1/2"-thick jalapeño slice, with seeds

6 ounces tequila Blanco

4 ounces simple syrup

2 ounces fresh lime juice

3 cups ice

Optional garnish: Watermelon wedges and sliced jalapeños

Directions:

Combine 3 1/2 cups watermelon pieces, frozen + 1/2"-thick jalapeño slice, with seeds + 6 ounces tequila Blanco + 4 ounces simple syrup + 2 ounces fresh lime juice + 3 cups ice optional garnish: Watermelon wedges and sliced jalapeños.

Cook's NoteHead to the farmers' market for peak-season fruit. Freeze the fruit in a single layer on a parchment-lined baking sheet until solid. Purée ingredients in a blender until smooth and very thick. Divide among glasses and serve.

Cold Facts:

The drier the ice, the better. Melting ice makes for a watery cocktail.

No need to upgrade your blender. The old one will do the trick just fine.

Texture Matters:

Frozen drinks should look too thick when poured into the glass. They will loosen immediately.

Watermelon Margarita Ice Pops

Preparation time: 10 minutes

Servings: 2

Ingredients:

5 cups chopped seedless watermelon (1 1/4 pounds)

2 tablespoons fresh lime juice

3 tablespoons superfine granulated sugar

1/4 cup water

1/4 cup silver tequila

Equipment: 8 (1/3-cup) ice pop molds and 8 wooden sticks

0 and 8 wooden sticks

Directions:

Purée all ingredients in a blender until smooth, then strain through a fine-mesh sieve into a large measuring cup, pressing on and then discarding solids.

Skim off any foam, then pour into molds. Freeze for 30 minutes. Insert sticks, then freeze until firm, about 24 hours.

Watermelon Margaritas

Preparation time: 10 minutes

Servings: 4

Ingredients:

2 cups cubed seeded watermelon

2 cups crushed ice

1/3 cup tequila

1/4 cup white sugar

1/4 cup lime juice

1 tablespoon vodka

1 tablespoon orange liqueur

Directions:

Combine watermelon, ice, tequila, sugar, lime juice, vodka, and orange liqueur in a blender; blend well. Pour margaritas into glasses.

Watermelon Refresher

Preparation time: 10 minutes

Servings: 10

Ingredients:

10 cups diced seeded watermelon

1/2 cup water

1/3 cup agave nectar

1 1/2 cups tequila (such as Patron®)

1 cup frozen blueberries

1 sprig of mint leaves, for garnish

Directions:

Blend the watermelon in a blender until smooth; pour into a large pitcher.

Stir the water and agave nectar together in a small bowl; add to the watermelon. Stir the tequila into the watermelon mixture. Add the blueberries and garnish with the mint to serve.

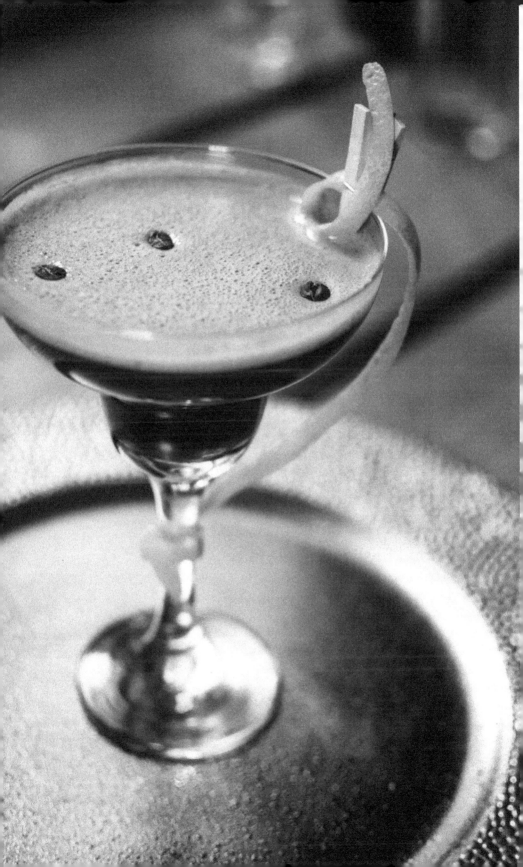

Rum Keto Cocktails

Pineapple Caipirinhas

Preparation time: 15 minutes

Servings: 8

Ingredients:

400ml light rum. You can also use Cachaca Liqueur instead

800ml fresh pineapple juice

1 pineapple, cut into chunks

A few sprigs of mint

8 tbsp caster sugar

The juice of 4 limes

Crushed ice

Directions:

Take a large pitcher and add around half the pineapple chunks, mint, lime juice, and the sugar

Use the end of a rolling pin to mash the mixture down into a pulp

Add the rum or cachaca and combine with the pulp

Add the pineapple juice to the top of the pitcher

Take 8 glasses and add some crushed ice into each

Pour the cocktail into the glasses equally

Use any left-over pineapple to decorate the glasses

Mojito cocktail

Preparation time: 10 minutes

Servings: 2

Ingredients:

3mint leaves

Mint spring

2ml white rum¾ Fresh lime juice

½ simple syrup

Club soda

Lime wheel

Directions:

Pour the mint into a shaker

Add the rum, lime juice, simple syrup together with ice and shake it for a while.

Strain it on highball glass over fresh ice

Add club soda, garnish with mint and lime wheel

The Goombay Smash

Preparation time: 10 minutes

Servings: 2

Ingredients:

Ice cubes

Pineapple juice (6 tbsp)

Orange juice (1/4 cup)

Coconut-flavored rum (1/4 cup)

Rum (2 tbsp, light)

Rum (2 tbsp, gold)

Dark rum (2 tbsp)

Pineapple (2 wedges)

Orange (2 slices)

Directions:

In a cocktail shaker, add the orange juice, all rums, and pineapple juice.

Cover tightly and shake until it becomes very cold. Fill 2 medium glasses with ice.

Strain over the cocktail mixture ensuring to divide equally. Garnish with orange slices and pineapple wedges.

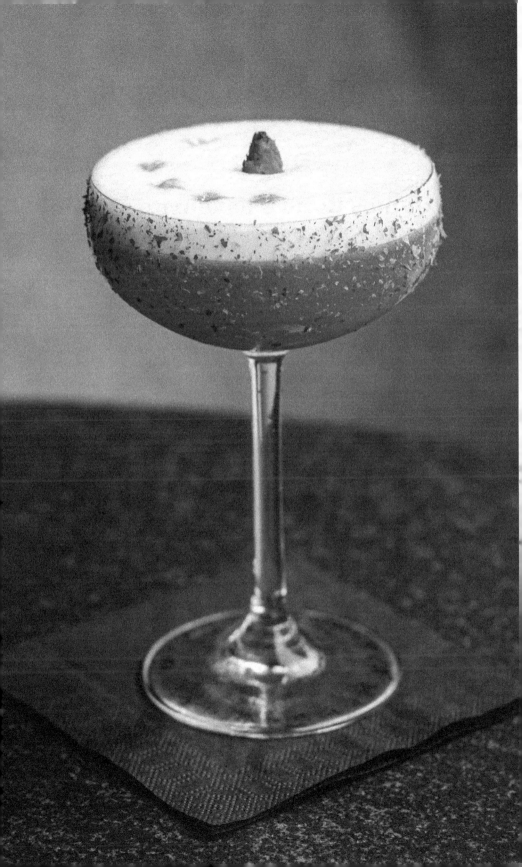

Vodka Keto Cocktails

James Bond's Favourite Martini

Preparation time: 10 minutes

Servings: 1

Ingredients:

1 tbsp vermouth, the dry version is best for this cocktail

60ml vodka

Peel of a lemon for decoration

Directions:

Take a jug and combine the vermouth and vodka with some ice

Pour into a cocktail shaker and give it a few good shakes

Use a strainer to pour the cocktail into a martini glass

Decorate with the lemon peel

The Sunset Over Waterloo

Preparation time: 10 minutes

Servings: 1

Ingredients:

100ml schnapps, peach works best for this cocktail

200ml vanilla flavored vodka

A little grenadine to taste

500ml peach juice, chilled

A little lemonade

A handful of fresh or frozen raspberries

A handful of ice cubes

Directions:

Take a mixing jug and add the vodka, juice, and schnapps, combining well

Pour the cocktail evenly between 8 glasses

Add a few ice cubes to each glass and fill up to the top with lemonade

Take a teaspoon and pour a little of the grenadine over the spoon, into the glass

Decorate with the raspberries

Apple & Ginger Vodka Punch

Preparation time: 10 minutes

Servings: 8

Ingredients:

500ml apple juice

500ml vanilla flavored vodka

1 liter ginger beer

The juice of 2 limes

2 limes sliced into wedges

1 thinly sliced apple

A small piece of peeled and sliced ginger

Directions:

Take a large jug and add all the liquid ingredients, combining well

Add the ginger, wedges of lime, and the apple to the jug and mix once more

Add ice to your glasses and pour the cocktail over the ice

Chocolate Orange Vodka

Preparation time: 10 minutes

Servings: 5

Ingredients:

100ml vodka

100ml creme de cacao

60ml orange liqueur

40ml fresh orange juice

100g caster sugar

The zest of 1 large orange

100ml cold water

A handful of ice cubes

A little dark chocolate, grated, for decoration

Directions:

Take a small saucepan and combine the water with the sugar and orange zest. Allow to boil, stirring regularly

Allow the syrup to cool and strain into a small bowl

Take 4 cocktail glasses and wet the rims a little before dipping them into the grated chocolate for decoration. Place it to one side

Take a cocktail shaker and add the creme de cacao, vodka, orange juice, and the stained syrup you just made

Add the ice and shake

Pour into the prepared glasses

Floral Prosecco & Vodka Cocktail

Preparation time: 10 minutes

Servings: 4

Ingredients:

100ml vodka

300ml Prosecco

25ml ginger beer or cordial

The juice of 1 orange

The juice of 1 lemon

A few hibiscus flower, including the syrup

A handful of ice cubes

Directions:

Take a cocktail shaker and combine the lemon juice, orange juice, vodka, and ginger, with a little ice

Take 4 champagne glasses and add a hibiscus flower inside each one

Use a strainer to pour the cocktail into each glass, leaving space for the Prosecco

Add a little Prosecco to each glass

Top with a teaspoon of the hibiscus syrup

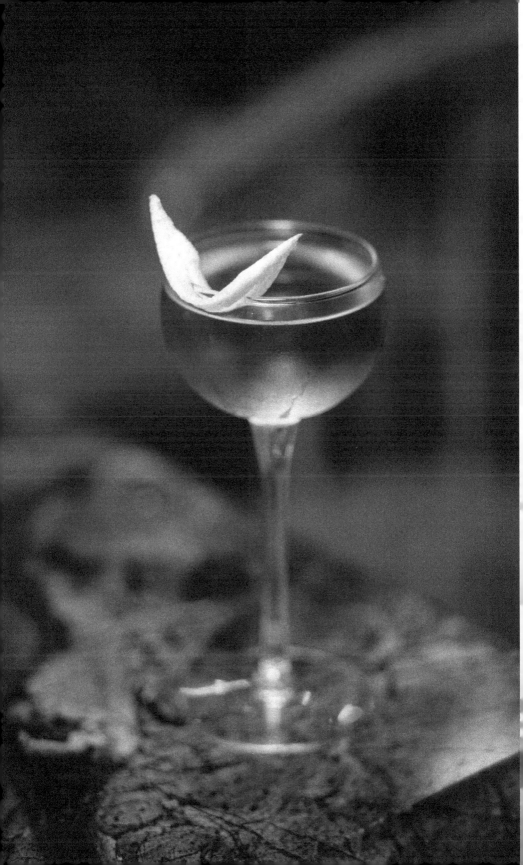

Keto Liqueurs

Chocolate liqueur

Preparation time: 30 minutes

Servings: 3

Ingredients:

26.4oz. of whole milk

8.8oz. of sugar

8.8oz. of fresh liquid cream

5.3oz. of pure alcohol

3.5oz. of bitter cocoa powder

3.5oz. of dark chocolate

Directions:

To prepare Chocolate Liqueur, start by combining the milk and cream in a large saucepan. Add the sugar and begin to heat the mixture. Also, add the cocoa beginning immediately to mix with the whisk to avoid the formation of lumps. Continuing to stir with the whisk, slowly bring to a boil.

Let it simmer for about 10 minutes, continuing to stir; then add the coarsely chopped chocolate.

Mix carefully until it melts. Turn off the heat and let it cool. Finally, add the alcohol and mix well.

Filter the mixture through a narrow mesh strainer to avoid any residual lumps. Once completely cooled, distribute the chocolate liqueur in clean and completely dry bottles. Close the bottles tightly and let the liqueur mature for 20-30 days before consumption, so that the flavor of the alcohol is softer and less intensive.

Tips:

The bottled chocolate liqueur can be kept in the pantry for about 90 days. It is recommended to wait at least 20 days before enjoying it, because just after **Directions:** it will be heavily alcoholic.

Flower Martini

Preparation time: 10 minutes

Servings: 2

Ingredients:

8 milliliters rose water

15 milliliters cold water

15 milliliters dry vermouth

15 milliliters elderflower liqueur

60 milliliters London dry gin

Directions:

Stir ingredients with ice and strain into chilled glass.
Garnish using a rose petal.

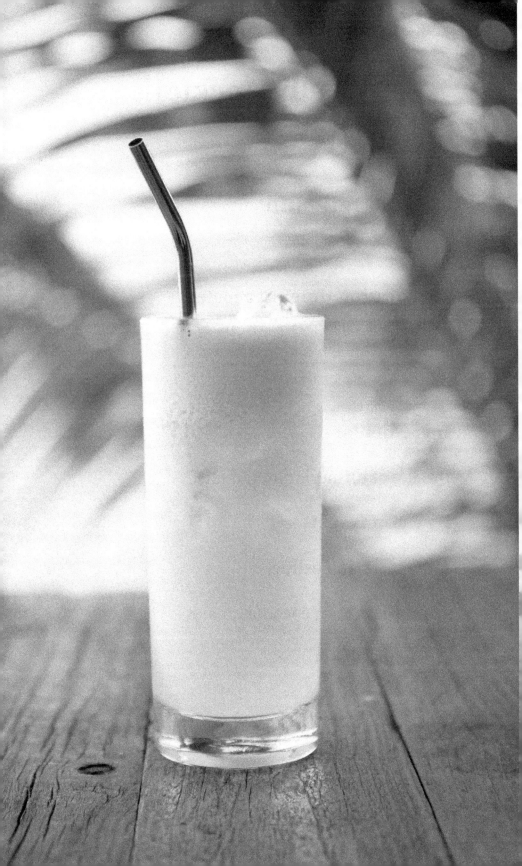

Keto Mocktails

Mocktail chai

Preparation time: 10 minutes

Servings: 4

Ingredients:

1/2 cup of turmeric almond juice

1/2 cup of Ceylon tea

1/2 tsp. almond extract

3/4 cup cream or coconut cream

Cinnamon stick

Directions:

Pour all the ingredients into a serving glass. Mix until combined.

Garnish with a cinnamon stick.

Lemon with coconut

Preparation time: 10 minutes

Servings: 4

Ingredients:

1/2 cup of coconut water

1/2 cup of tonic water, chilled

1 tablespoon. lime juice

pinch of rosemary for garnish

lime zest for garnish

Directions:

Pour all the ingredients into a serving glass. Mix until combined.

Garnish with spiral lime, rosemary, and lime zest.

Pomegranate twist

Preparation time: 10 minutes

Servings: 4

Ingredients:

1/2 cup of sparkling water

1/4 cup pomegranate juice com

Ice

Orange zest for garnish

Directions:

In a glass, add ice and pour all the ingredients.

Mix and garnish with a fresh orange twist.

Pomegranate-Lemon Spritzer

Preparation time: 10 minutes

Servings: 4

Ingredients:

1 bottle (16 ounces) pomegranate juice

1 (2-liter) bottle club soda, unflavored sparkling water, or lemon-lime soda

1 cup fresh lemon juice (8 to 10 large lemons)

½ to ¾ cup sugar (to taste)

Directions:

In a large pitcher, combine pomegranate juice, lemon juice, and enough water or soda to fill the pitcher. Add sugar 1 tablespoonful at a time, tasting frequently, until desired sweetness is reached (see Note).

Serve immediately, over ice if desired.

Note:

You may find, especially if you use lemon-lime soda, that this drink is sweet enough without added sugar.

Red moon

Preparation time: 10 minutes

Servings: 4

Ingredients:

180 ml of carbonated water

60 ml of plum-cinnamon shrub

Plum slices to decorate

Directions:

Mix the shrub with the carbonated water in a glass filled with ice and mix well. Garnish with plum slices.

Thai mango ice tea

Preparation time: 10 minutes

Servings: 4

Ingredients:

2 teaspoons of cashew drink

2 teaspoons of condensed milk

2 teaspoons of granulated sugar

½ teaspoon of molasses

1 bag of Thai black tea

240 ml of boiling water

4 slices of dehydrated mango and a few more cut into thin strips to decorate

Directions:

In a large cup or bowl, steep the tea, mango, and sugar in hot water, then allow to cool. Remove the mango and the teabag. Add the remaining ingredients and mix. Serve in a large glass filled with ice cubes and garnish with the thin mango strips.

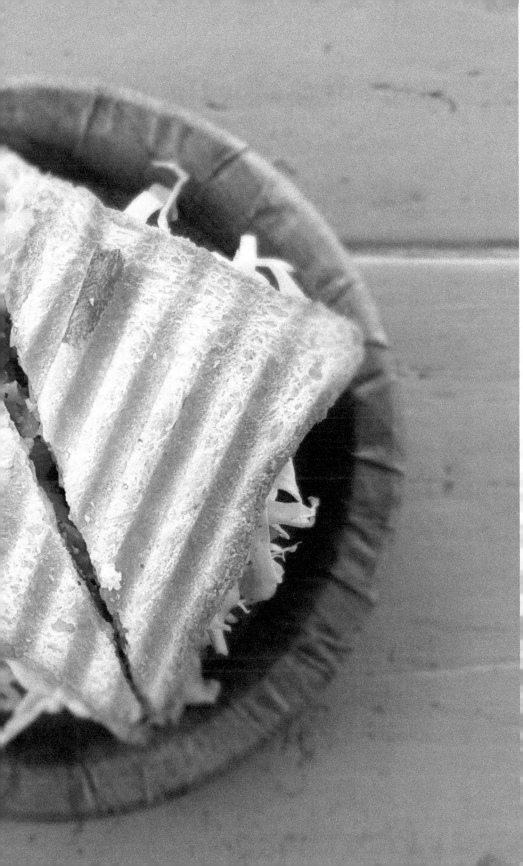

Keto Snacks for Happy Hour

Low Carb BBQ Sauce

Preparation time: 10 minutes

Cooking Time: 5 minutes

Servings: 1-16 ounces

Ingredients:

1/4 cup of Lecanto Gold dark colored sugar substitute OR sugar of your choice

1/4 cup of apple juice vinegar

1/4 cup of white vinegar

1/2 cup of water

2 tablespoons of genuine spread

1 can tomato paste

1 teaspoon of garlic powder

1 teaspoon of onion powder

1 teaspoon of dry yellow mustard

1 teaspoon of salt

1 teaspoon of cayenne pepper (discretionary)

1 teaspoon of fluid smoke (discretionary)

Directions:

If you like a thinner sauce, add more water until desired thickness is achieved.

If you like an increasingly acrid sauce, add more vinegar.

Go simple with the fluid smoke, a little is enough!

This formula is effectively versatile to various sugars. Utilizing white sugar will bring about an increasingly red sauce.

The margarine makes a pleasant lustrous completion and makes the sauce be on whatever you brush it on.

Nutrition: calories 355, fat 28, fiber 2, carbs 6, protein 37

Tzatziki

Preparation time: 10 minutes

Cooking Time: 0 minutes

Servings: 8 servings

Ingredients:

½ c shredded cucumber, drained.

1 tsp. salt

1 T olive oil

1 T fresh mint finely chopped.

2 garlic cloves

1 c full-fat Greek yogurt

1 t lemon juice

Directions:

Place shredded cucumber on a strainer for an hour or squeeze out moisture through a cheesecloth.

Mix all ingredients in a medium bowl.

Refrigerate.

Use as a vegetable dip, a dip for dehydrated vegetables, or a sauce for lamb, beef, or chicken. It is also a perfect accompaniment for fried summer squash.

Nutrition: calories 210, fat 8, fiber 2, carbs 8, protein 7

Caprese Snack Pizza

Preparation time: 10 minutes

Cooking Time: 20 minutes

Servings: 4

Ingredients:

½ cup cheddar cheese, shredded

1 cup tomatoes, sliced

½ cup fresh mozzarella, sliced

¼ cup fresh basil, chopped

1 tablespoon balsamic vinegar

Directions:

Lightly oil a small or medium-sized skillet.

Place the cheddar cheese in the skillet over medium heat, and spread it around to form an even, circular layer.

Reduce the heat to medium-low and cook until the edges of the cheese are crisp and browned for approximately 2-3 minutes.

Carefully remove the cheese "crust" from the pan and slide it onto a plate.

Top the crust with basil, tomatoes, and mozzarella.

Drizzle with balsamic vinegar, and cut it into wedges before serving.

Nutrition: calories 355, fat 28, fiber 2, carbs 6, protein 37

Asiago Chive Chips

Preparation time: 10 minutes

Cooking Time: 20 minutes

Servings: 4

Ingredients:

1 cup Asiago cheese, shredded

1 tablespoon fresh chives, chopped

½ teaspoon salt

½ teaspoon black pepper

Directions:

Preheat the oven to 350°F and line a baking sheet with parchment paper.

In a bowl, combine the Asiago cheese, chives, salt, and black pepper.

Place spoonfuls of the cheese mixture onto the baking sheet, leaving enough room for the cheese to spread out as it bakes.

Place the baking sheet in the oven and bake for 3-5 minutes, or until crisp and browned.

Remove the pan from the oven and let it cool before carefully removing the chips with a spatula.

Nutrition: calories 354, fat 14, fiber 2, carbs 16, protein 26

Extra Creamy Easy Guacamole

Preparation time: 10 minutes

Cooking Time: 20 minutes

Servings: 4

Ingredients:

2 avocados

½ cup cream cheese, softened

½ cup jarred salsa

¼ cup fresh cilantro

2 teaspoons lime juice

1 teaspoon salt

1 teaspoon black pepper

Directions:

Peel and pit the avocados, and place them with the cream cheese in a bowl or food processor. Blend until creamy.

Add the jarred salsa, cilantro, and lime juice. Season with salt and black pepper as desired and mix well.

Serve immediately or cover tightly and refrigerate until ready to serve.

Nutrition: calories 210, fat 8, fiber 2, carbs 8, protein 7

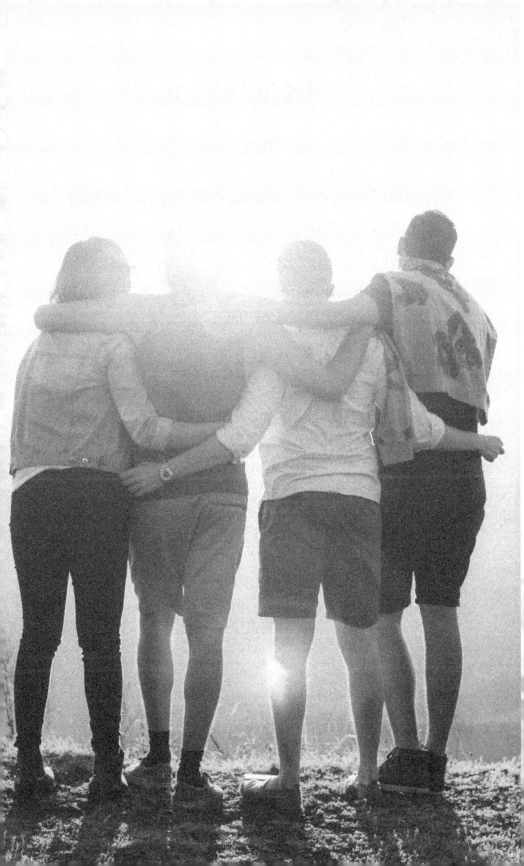

Conclusion

Congratulations on making it to the end of this keto cocktail book. My keto cocktails recipes are famous for being really tasty but also healthy, their properties have beneficial effects on our health and prevent certain types of diseases and offer the certainty of losing weight. Thanks to these healthy and delicious drinks, our lifestyle will change positively and our body will purify itself. I am sure that all the drinks we made have entertained you and satisfied you.

Good luck.

CPSIA information can be obtained
at www.ICGtesting.com
Printed in the USA
BVHW061241020621
608544BV00005B/1521

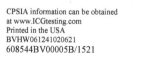

9 781802 893397